Promises Promises

Hello and thanks for purchasing my book!

Before we get started, I'm going to make a couple of promises to you...

Promise #1: If you read this book, you will know the value of maintaining truly normal blood sugars. There are many benefits but the most important ... halting the progression of the disease and thereby halting the progression of diabetic complications.

Promise #2: I will show you concrete, actionable steps to start reducing your blood sugars today!

There are two types of people in this world...

People who know they need to obtain and maintain truly normal blood sugars ... and those who do not know.

Sadly millions will never know the truth and will suffer from diabetic complications until they pass away.

If you don't already, you will soon learn the importance of maintaining truly normal, non-diabetic blood sugars.

Steve Cooksey
Author and Founder
diabetes-warrior.net

D1188362

1

Preface

Testimonial by Karen Gale. (Thank you Karen!)

Before I began my journey, my health was quickly spiraling downward.

I am a type 2 diabetic who was battling:

- high blood sugar
- high triglycerides and high cholesterol
- severe migraines
- high blood pressure
- other ailments including acid reflux, allergies, etc.

I thought this was how I'd be living the rest of my life until I met Steve Cooksey. He introduced me to a low carb, paleo lifestyle that was life changing!

Within 3 months, I quickly reduced prescription medications and 1.5 years later I was prescription drug free!

Diabetes goes back many generations in my family as do the side effects of amputations and blindness. To be a diabetic and reduce medications was unheard of in my family; I am the first to do so!

Not only do I experience truly normal blood sugars, but I also experience a high amount of energy as well. I incorporate exercise into my daily routine. Initially I started with water aerobics and worked my way up to cross fit boot camps.

Over the past 4.5 years, I've lost over 40 pounds, going from a size 14 to 6 in clothes. I encourage you to read this book; it can change your life!

Karen Gale

Thriving, not just surviving.

Congratulations for taking the first step to better health!

Since 2009 I have been THRIVING! ... and I want you to thrive too! I wrote this book hoping to inspire all diabetics to maintain truly normal blood sugars!

Why do I want you to have truly normal blood sugars?

To halt the progression of diabetes and the progression of diabetic complications!

Steve Note: Notice I didn't say that I want you to have 'normal diabetic blood sugars' or even normal prediabetic blood sugars... no, I want YOU to have truly normal, non-diabetic blood sugars.

When I tell diabetics the message above ... many look at me in disbelief, or even worse laugh in my face. Trust me on this, YOU can do it. I know because I and many others have done it too.

There is a better way to self-treat diabetes!

I urge you to 'read and heed' the contents of this book, it absolutely can change your life. It changed my life and the lives of many others.

The vast majority of diabetics suffer from diabetic complications because they maintain elevated blood sugars. Before you can maintain truly normal blood sugars, **you must first learn how to reduce your blood sugars, and then learn how to maintain normal ranges.**

Cause of Type 2 Diabetes is Insulin Resistance

Type 2 Diabetes is a disease of insulin resistance. It doesn't just happen overnight, the damage takes years, even decades to manifest itself.

Reducing the body's requirements for insulin is a major way to improve your health and fitness. This can be accomplished by reducing insulin requirements using a very low carb diet and by increasing demand for glucose with weight resistance exercise.

By the end of this book, you will know exactly what you need to do, to start improving your insulin resistance and reducing your blood sugars.

Book Reviews

I wrote this book originally in 2014, five years into my diabetes journey. Through the years I've received a lot of feedback about this book improving the lives of people and I just wanted to give you a 'taste' of the book reviews I've received.

By the way, this my 3rd edition (2022), I like to update the book when new research or news comes available.

Note: I didn't write this book to be a complete A-Z manuscript for diabetes care.

I set out to write a short, to the point book, that someone could easily read in a day.

More importantly, I wanted to write a book a person could begin to implement immediately to reduce blood sugars ... today.

"If you are a diabetic or maybe just have blood sugar issues, you need to read this."

"This book took no time at all to read and I gained a lot from it. It was simple and straight to the point. I think the diet concepts were simple to understand and simple to implement. Simple really. Did I mention simple? If you need to control blood sugar levels start here."

"Great information. It is a short, to the point book. For $5 it is a slam dunk, get it. Too many times I buy health books and find that they spend too much time repeating what has already been said and could summarize everything in 20 pages.

One negative review states that everything in the book can be found on his blog, which is true but how that is a negative is beyond me. The writer's blog documents his journey to solve type II diabetes and he spells out what he has done. ..."

Disclaimer: Who Am I Not?

I am NOT a doctor, nutritionist, nor diabetes educator. In fact, I have ZERO medical training and NO formal nutritional training. However, I am a diabetic who follows his own 'diabetic diet' (backed by scientific research) and has normal blood glucose while taking -0- drugs and -0- insulin.

If I can figure this out, why can't the Medical Industry?

Greed?
Intellectual Laziness?
Willful Ignorance?

(And I see this as a huge advantage, I wasn't biased by the failed protocols and biased research of the past.)

Who I Am

I am a formerly obese, formerly drug and insulin dependent diabetic who has been diabetic drug and insulin free since 2009!

Below, my 'before and after' pictures. The picture on the left was December 2008, a few months before the wheels literally fell off of my health 'wagon'.

A few months later, I would be diagnosed with diabetes and my life would change forever.

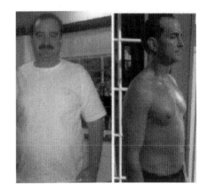

The picture on the right is from November 2009, roughly 9 months after a diabetes diagnosis.

I look pretty much the same today, just 13 years older... and meaner.

Think about this for a moment... How many diabetics have weaned off all drugs AND insulin... and maintained truly normal blood sugars and normal weight for 13 years!?

Not ONLY am I diabetes drug and insulin free, I am medical industry services free!

That's my way of saying that I haven't been to the doctor or any 'medical industry professional' for diabetes or sickness, since 2009!

At my diagnosis I was taking (4) insulin shots a day!!! ... just to survive. But I quickly weaned off all drugs and insulin... my 'rebirth' began almost immediately as I began to research the best diets and best lifestyles to self-treat diabetes.

Since 2009, I've read and researched everything I could get my hands on.

Not only have I read and researched, I've done many experiments through the years...

- High carb, moderate and low carb
- Lower fat, high fat, low fat
- Low protein, adequate protein and even high protein
- Intense anaerobic exercise vs aerobic exercise
- Fasting including water-only, fat-fasts, etc
- Supplements, chromium, cinnamon, iodine, etc.
- Self-experimentation is a major reason for my successful self-treatment of diabetes.

Some experiments are shared: http://www.diabetes-warrior.net.

Conversations with my Doctor

I respect my doctor, I haven't seen him since 2009... but I respect and appreciate him. I'll just share three quick conversations from the months after my diabetes diagnosis.

1. At diagnosis, a few days after exiting the hospital, he didn't push the high carb, grain-based 'diabetes diet' on me, the hospital nutritionist and diabetes educator had already done that.

   It didn't make sense... "eat the same foods I was eating, just less of them".

My doctor knew I was researching and he suggested a 'low glycemic' diet and suggested I look into it. I bought the book, and while I don't recommend it ... it did lead me down the path of self-experimentation and self-discovery.

The lower I ate in carbs... the less drugs and insulin I needed.

2. Several weeks later I had a follow up, and my blood sugars were much improved.

   Still on diabetes drugs and insulin, but my blood sugars were often in 'normal range' but solidly 'prediabetic'... and no longer diabetic levels.

   He knew too that I was cranking down the carbs, losing weight, feeling better...

   He said the words that I will **NEVER** forget. (and I get goosebumps every time I think of them).

   "You are doing great Steve, keep it up. We have a diabetes nutrition class next week but I don't think you need to go... you could probably teach the class."

   ... I declined the invitation.

3. Another conversation that I will never forget... the day I informed my doctor that I had stopped insulin and drugs ... without checking with him first.

   This was at my next follow up, 1 ½ months after diagnosis. About a week before the appointment I'd stopped taking all drugs... drugs for diabetes, hypertension, cholesterol...

8

Why? Because by then my blood sugars were in normal ranges. I stopped all the drugs and all the insulin shots. I was FREE!

When I told my doctor his jaw tightened a bit. He looked through my chart flipping pages, and then said...

 "You should never stop taking drugs without checking with me first. But I've got to say, I think you did the right thing. I wouldn't change what you are doing. Keep it up."

And so I did...

I've been 'keeping it up' for 13 years... and I'm never going to stop researching and experimenting.

I'm NEVER going back to the way I used to eat, play ... or live!

Why do I say, "I found a better way to self-treat diabetes"? ... and what does it mean when I say I "thrive"?

1. Weaned off all drugs and insulin

2. Obtained and maintained truly normal blood sugars

3. Lost and maintained an 80 lb weight loss

4. Halted the progression of known diabetic complications

Since 2009, I've devoted my life to not only continuing to seek out the very best diabetic care practices but also the best ways to add years to my life ... and add more LIVING to those years!

What About You?

What's your diabetes story? How will it end?

I've given you my 'diabetes story'. Unlike the typical diabetic, diabetes was actually a blessing for me. It made me focus on eating a truly healthy and low carb diet. It pushed me to exercise and get outside to enjoy the sun and nature.

Before I implemented the changes in this book... I was sick and tired, of being sick and tired.

What's your reason for wanting to reduce your blood sugars?

For most diabetics, they just want to live a normal life without the anxiety and worry of a life filled with the pain and anguish of diabetic complications... neuropathy, organ failures, amputations, etc.

How will your diabetes story end?

With the information in this book... you too can have a happy ending, you too can rekindle a ZEST FOR LIVING!

You too can live out the rest of your years without the fear of diabetic complications and the debilitating progression of the disease.

In large diabetes groups, every day I see the signs of anguish, pain and suffering... and it's almost all needless.

And as I'll show you, the ADA and the Medical Industry are responsible for much of the pain and suffering. Yes, personal responsibility has a role to play, but before we can blame diabetics, they need to be given accurate and healthy information.

Find Your Biggest Why

You need to know 'the why' ... why you want to improve your blood sugars.

The obvious answer is, 'for better health'. But I want you to dig deeper, and think of concrete and specific reasons why you want better health.

- Do you want to enjoy the rest of your life without the worry of diabetic complications?

- Do you want to travel and lead an active lifestyle with your spouse?

- Do you want to watch your children marry and start a family?

Whatever the reason or the 'why'... find them, write them down and place them in several locations... at work, at home on the refrigerator and inside the door of cabinets or cupboards.

Spend a few more dollars and have them laminated, hand them out to your friends, relatives and co-workers, especially those you may eat lunch with. These steps are of course optional, but if you think you may 'cheat' and fall off the wagon, taking extra precautions is never a bad thing.

Let everyone know that you have made changes in your life and that you want their help.

Work the plan and let it work for you.

Your body will love you for it.

What is Diabetes?

Diabetes is a disease of elevated blood sugars...

To be diagnosed with diabetes (or prediabetes) you have to surpass the threshold approved by the medical industry.

Here are the latest thresholds approved by the American Diabetes Association in their latest 2022 version of Diabetes Care Guidelines.
Take a good look at these numbers, I'll be using them often.

Normal non-diabetic fasting blood sugars are **70-99 mg/dl** (3.8 - 5.5 mmol/l) and a **normal A1C is below 5.7**.

Abnormal Blood Sugars are 100+ mg/dl (5.6 mmol/l) and an A1C of 5.7 or higher.

Overnight Fasting Blood Sugars and A1C

	mg/dl	mmol/l	A1C
Normal	70-99	3.8 - 5.5	Below 5.7
Prediabetic	100-125	5.6 - 6.9	5.7 - 6.4
Diabetic	126+	7.0+	6.5 or above

Steve Note: I don't agree with the thresholds, but for now we'll use these numbers. I think they should be even lower. Studies show that EVEN slightly elevated but still within the normal range of blood sugars can over time, lead to diabetic complications.

I include studies supporting this in the Addendum section at the end of the book.

Do you want truly normal blood sugars? Or do you want **ABNORMAL** blood sugars?

I hope you are saying... "I want truly normal blood sugars!"

Blood Sugar Confusion

There is so much confusion regarding diabetic blood sugar targets.

It would take another book to debunk all of the fake news in the diabetes world... but one of the SINGLE biggest misconceptions is **Truly Normal Blood Sugar** levels.

We know from the chart that normal fasting blood sugars are below 100 mg/dl (5.5 mmol/l), yet so many diabetics do not know this one simple fact.

So many diabetics think an A1C of 6.0, 6.5 or even 7.0 is 'ok' or 'just fine' because their doctor said so.

I know why diabetics believe these harmful falsehoods (lies) ... it's because the ADA and the Medical Industry do not tell diabetics the truth.

If you don't believe me... keep reading, I prove this to you later in the book.

Normal Diabetic Vs Truly Normal Blood Sugars

The ADA and the Medical Industry mix and match words like 'normal diabetic blood sugars' vs 'diabetic recommendations' vs 'diabetic targets' vs 'diabetic goals'.

It can be quite confusing for even the most veteran diabetics … much less the newly diagnosed. I devote sections to the book to break these down in detail, but for now just know that they are not the same.

When I say, 'normal blood sugars' … I mean truly normal blood sugars.

The secret to living diabetic complication free is truly normal blood sugars.

I didn't say the secret is **prediabetic blood sugar levels**. I didn't say the secret was to maintain **diabetic blood sugar levels** …

This is an important distinction and it is a distinction you are NOT likely to hear from your doctor, nutritionist or diabetes educator.

ADA Blood Sugar Targets

Ok, we know 'truly' normal fasting blood sugars are below 100 mg/dl (5.5 mmol/l), now let's look at the Medical Industry and ADA Blood Sugar Targets.

I decided soon after a diabetes diagnosis that I wanted truly normal blood sugars. Sadly thanks to both of my diabetic grandmothers I knew the pain, suffering and anxiety caused by elevated blood sugars.

Collectively my grandmothers (one a type 1, the other a type 2) had strokes, heart attacks, neuropathy, retinopathy, heart disease, and amputations.

I knew where the standard diabetic 'road' would lead, and I vowed to fight the disease.

It sounds corny now, but as a 47 year old laying in the Intensive Care Unit as a newly diagnosed diabetic... I told myself, **"I was too young to die old"**, and I vowed to fight this disease... and I did.

It was a no-brainer for me as a diabetic to seek normal blood sugars, who wouldn't do everything they could to halt the progression of the disease?

It's apparently not so obvious to those who profit from diabetes... doctors, nutritionists, dietitians and diabetes educators.

Odd isn't it? The people who profit from the ravages of diabetes, namely the ADA, Big Food, Big Pharma and the Medical Industry promote harmful targets AND a High Carb diet that makes obtaining Truly Normal Blood Sugars nearly impossible.

ADA A1C Recommendation

From the previous sections, we know that at least according to the ADA an A1C below 5.7 is considered 'normal'. I took that information directly from their site.

So if you had to guess, what would you think the ADA's A1C target or recommendation would be?

If you guessed 'below 5.7" ... you would be wrong.

Below is the ADA's A1C Recommendation for diabetics ... from this page on the ADA's site.

Recommendations

> **6.5a** An A1C goal for many nonpregnant adults of
>
> <7% (53 mmol/mol) without significant hypoglycemia
>
> is appropriate. **A**

Why does the ADA recommend blood sugar targets that **DO NOT** prevent the progression of the disease and that does NOT prevent the horrible pain and suffering caused by diabetic complications?

The ADA does recommend blood sugar targets that guarantees the progression of the disease and guarantees pain and suffering from diabetic complications!

Isn't that incredible? Why would they NOT recommend truly normal blood sugars? The ADA's policies cause so much pain and suffering.

The ADA knows every diabetic should obtain and maintain truly normal blood sugars to escape the ravages of diabetes and diabetic complications ... yet they promote targets that cause harm.

I won't attempt to answer the 'why?' question now ... but my guess is that it has to do with pleasing their largest corporate donors and diabetes bedfellows ... Big Food, Big Pharma and the Medical Industry.

A Truthful Graphic From the ADA

The ADA doesn't promote truly normal blood sugars but they provide hints, like this graphic below.

Reminder: From the ADA, A1C of 5.7 and above is prediabetes and an A1C above 6.5 is the threshold for diabetes.

However from this graphic below, we can see that even in the higher ranges of 'Normal" there is yellow or caution long before 5.7 and there is definitely red or a danger zone in the prediabetic range, long before the blood sugar levels get to be official diabetic levels.

This graphic tells more of the truth than the ADA has ever stated or written.

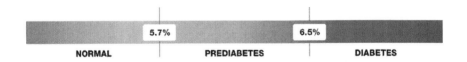

This graphic can be found on the ADA website here.

ADA's Pre and Post Meal Blood Sugar Targets

Remember fasting blood sugars over 100 mg/dl (5.5 mmol/l) and A1C's over 5.7 are considered **ABNORMAL** by the Medical Industry and cause long term harm.

... but what about pre and post meal blood sugars?

The next table is directly from the ADA's website, (source link).

Table 6.3—Summary of glycemic recommendations for many nonpregnant adults with diabetes	
A1C	<7.0% (53 mmol/mol)*#
Preprandial capillary plasma glucose	80–130 mg/dL* (4.4–7.2 mmol/L)
Peak postprandial capillary plasma glucose†	<180 mg/dL* (10.0 mmol/L)

We've already talked about the harmful ADA A1C recommendation of less than 7, so I'll just address the preprandial (before meal) and the peak postprandial (after meal) blood sugar recommendations chart from the previous page.

- **Pre Meal Target:** The ADA promotes blood sugars all the way up to **130 mg/dl (7.2 mmol/l)** as being within the desired target range recommendations!!!

  Imagine a typical diabetic eating the usual high carb diet of 60 grams of carbs per meal ... what is going to happen to their blood sugars?! They will SOAR into even higher ranges.

  Before a meal, a diabetic's blood sugar should be normal,

19

less than 100 mg/dl (5.5 mmol/l).
That should be the target, the goal, and the
recommendation... end of story.

How can you win the war against diabetes with the wrong
goals, targets, or recommendations? You can't and the ADA
knows it.

The targets are shameful, even more so when the ADA
promotes a high carb diet. Their targets and diet do not
benefit diabetics, but they do benefit the ADA's largest
contributors with increased profits, namely... Big Food, Big
Pharma, and the Medical Industry.

- **Post Meal Target:** 180 mg/dl (10.0 mmol/l) is more
  harmful advice.

  As we already know, **180 mg/dl is a harmful
  recommendation**. But consider this, the ADA's Pre Meal
  Blood Sugar target is as high as 130 mg/dl.

  Suggesting that the typical obese, carb addicted diabetic
  could eat 60 grams of carbs as the ADA advocates, and stay
  below EVEN 180 mg/dl is ridiculous.

  An appropriate target would be to have blood sugars return
  back to pre meal levels ... which should be below 100 mg/dl
  (5.5 mmol/l).

  I'm not saying you should NEVER go above 100 mg/dl (5.5
  mmol/l) ... but I'm saying it should be brief and not chronic,
  like the vast majority of diabetics.

  For the medical industry and the ADA to claim that 180
  mg/dl (10.0 mmol/l) is within a desired range for
  diabetics... for anyone, is unethical and immoral, and

should be illegal.

THE GOAL should be TRULY NORMAL BLOOD SUGARS to halt the progression of the disease and to halt the resulting diabetic complications.

My Blood Sugar Targets

Our bodies were designed to operate within a tight range of blood sugar. If we exceed certain levels, insulin is secreted. If we go below certain levels our body produces glucose.

Why? Elevated blood sugars as well as low blood sugars are not healthy.

Here are my targets.

Overnight Fasting Blood Sugar Goals from 70 - 90 mg/dl (3.3 - 5.0 mmol/l)

If I could choose an overnight fasting number it would be 70 mg/dl (3.8 mmol/l).

Why?

 I could eat a low carb meal (as usual) and still stay in the 80's (4.4 - 5.3 mmol/l) after eating.

In the Addendum at the end of the book, I provide evidence (studies) as to why I set these specific blood sugar targets.

For now, I'm going to assume you agree and we will proceed.

Causes of Elevated Blood Sugar

The root cause of elevated blood sugars are insulin resistance and reduced pancreatic insulin production, there are other causes.

Potential Reasons for Elevated Blood Sugars

1. Carbohydrates in excess (including sugars and starches)
2. Dehydration
3. Lack of quality sleep
4. Stress
5. Illness, infections, injuries
6. Intense exercise
7. Drug interactions

Note: If you do not limit your carbohydrates you start the game already behind.

As you can see, there are factors other than carbohydrates that need to be considered if blood sugars remain elevated after adhering to the suggestions in this book.

To reduce your blood sugar levels

- limit total carbohydrates - to 30 grams or less per day
- stay hydrated
- get enough good quality sleep
- reduce stress with exercise, deep breathing, yoga, etc.
- sickness, infections or injuries need to be addressed
- exercise intensely only when blood sugars are not elevated
- research possible effects of drugs on blood sugar (and test with your meter)

The most important thing in the beginning is cutting carbs, work on all the other items above... but #1 is limiting carbs.

PhD in Me: Blood Sugar Testing

Everyone should have a blood sugar meter or glucometer for testing. I don't recommend relying only on a quarterly or even a monthly A1C.

1. Test new foods to see how they affect your blood sugars.

2. At a minimum you should test overnight fasting blood sugars as well as before meal, and 2 hours post meal.

3. To truly know the effect of a food or a meal on your blood sugars I suggest testing: Just before eating, 30 minutes after eating, 60 minutes after eating, 120 minutes after eating, and hourly until blood sugars return to the 'before' meal reading, which should be 100 mg/dl or less.

   Why do I suggest this protocol?

   Depending on the fat composition of the meal or food, there can be not only a delayed blood sugar reaction (spike) but also there can be an elongated response.

I know this is literally a 'pain' but if you follow my advice, soon you will be able to drastically reduce the amount of testing. "Today" I test my blood sugars about once or twice a month, unless I am experimenting.

It's to your benefit to become a 'self-scientist'... testing and recording the effects of foods and activities on your blood sugars. Which reminds me of the saying I've used in the past. "I've got a PhD in me."

Here's a post I wrote about the accuracy of meters. It's several years old now, but it will give you insights into different meters.

Note: As your blood sugars drop into truly normal blood sugars, you will need to reduce diabetes drugs and/or insulin. I did this myself, however talk to your doctor or diabetes educator about the reductions.

Eating to Reduce Blood Sugars

One of many myths we are led to believe: "You need to eat "X" amount of carbs per day".

It's a lie. You do not need to eat carbohydrates at all. Our liver makes all the glucose (sugar) our bodies need through the process called **gluconeogenesis**.

You must question everything!

If a doctor, nutritionist or diabetes educator tells me it is okay to eat something.... It means nothing to me. You should question the advice and test it with your meter... and I expect you to test my advice.

Any time you eat a new food that you haven't tested before, you should test your blood sugar.

Any time you eat a new food at a restaurant, you need to test. This is especially true for restaurant foods... even 'known' foods can have varying amounts of sugar added.
Learn to question everything, **every thing!** Especially if someone is profiting from the advice and make no mistake, everyone up and down the chain is profiting off of diabetics ... **every one**!

Nutritional Chart

On the next page is the nutritional chart that allowed me to go from an obese, drug and insulin dependent diabetic to a person of normal weight and truly normal blood sugar levels, all while weaning off drugs and insulin!

Note: Foods at and near the top should be eaten occasionally and in smaller amounts, namely fruits, berries and nuts. Foods below nuts can be eaten every day.

The main goal is to keep total carbohydrates below 30 grams per day.

*** As you reduce carbs, you may have to reduce medications (drugs, insulin, supplements) as blood sugars fall.

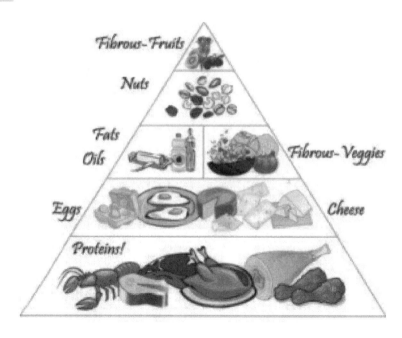

We'll talk about specific foods in more detail, but over the last several years, I typically eat between 5 - 15 grams of total carbohydrates per day and I exercise almost every day.

The reason I mention exercise now, so you will know that I have plenty of energy to exercise daily.

This meal plan is not just for diabetics. It is a meal plan I would encourage anyone to try, especially if they suffer from an illness, or take a drug.

KISS: Keep It Simple Stupid

There are a lot of different variations of 'diets' that one can choose when limiting carbohydrates, but there are two main variations. We will talk about both but I suggest #2, the "K.I.S.S. method.

1. **Count, measure and track your carbohydrates** making sure not to exceed 30 grams of total carbohydrates per day. I started using the 'count, measure and track' method... it works and it can work for you, but there is a better way... KISS.

2. K.I.S.S. - I suggest KISS when you first start.

   Simply eat meats, eggs, cheese, leafy green or fibrous vegetables until your blood sugars normalize.

   Note: KISS is the method I use today and have used for the last decade, except when I am experimenting with diet, etc.

   We'll talk more about the 'count, measure and track' method but now let's talk about KISS.

Why KISS?

Two main reasons.

1. It's so simple... anyone can do it.

2. You can start today! ... you can even start NOW!

Paralysis by Analysis

I see it all the time; people suffer from paralysis by analysis.

People believe they must learn everything about this way of eating before beginning! Every day they say, "ok, I'll start tomorrow." but something or someone always prevents them from starting.

Sadly 'tomorrow' never comes.

KISS: Simply eat meats, eggs, cheese, leafy green or fibrous vegetables until your blood sugars normalize.

Question my advice using your own blood sugar meter. Your blood sugars will trend down over the next week or two... your proof that it is working will be in your meter.

Do not use 'confusion' as an excuse not to start.

Yes, I get it, everyone is telling you to eat different things; I know it can be confusing. Remember I've been 'there', I truly do know how confusing it can be, but it doesn't have to be that way.

Trust your meter.

Eat the way I suggest for a couple of weeks. You have followed the advice of others and it has been a failure.

There is a better way to self-treat diabetes.

If you heed my advice, you will see amazing results. As you read the rest of this section just keep in mind, it all boils down to ... KISS.

Think about it, a handful of meat, a handful of fibrous vegetables, with a little cheese and an egg or two if you prefer...

It really could be THAT simple.

Purpose of the Diet

1 - Break the grain, sugar, carbohydrate addictions.

2 - Obtain and maintain normal blood sugar levels.

3 – Reach your weight-loss or fat-loss goals.

4 - Reduce the requirements and levels of insulin in the blood stream.

After accomplishing the points above, you can begin to add highER carb 'real foods' and see how your body handles them (optional). I added a few things back, usually as an experiment... but I always come back to 30 grams of carbs (or less) per day.

This meal plan works for all who try it and stick with it.

Work the plan and it will work for you!

A Meal Plan You Can "Live" With

This meal plan has worked for everyone who has tried it. If you work the plan... it will work for you! Remember to keep your carbohydrate totals below 30 grams per day and test new foods using your blood sugar meter!

Foods You Can EAT Every Day

Some people focus on foods they can never (or should never) eat again. That's a defeatist 'victim-creating' point of view.

I focus on all the wonderful, delicious and healthy foods that I **CAN** eat... every damn day if I choose.

Don't play the victim card to yourself. Soon you will be feeling better, being active... and enjoying life with a new sense of vigor. I sincerely tell people that a diabetes diagnosis saved my life! It can save your life too, if you embrace the new lifestyle.

I have made an attempt to cover at least all of the different types of foods. There are plenty of foods around the world not on this list, just remember ... limit carbs to 30 grams of total carbs per day.

Cronometer.com is an excellent free food dairy website and app. It's also great for looking up the protein, fat and carb totals of individual foods. I use it every day, not just for food... but for entering weight and blood sugar numbers.

Meats – beef, pork, poultry and fish. Meats are particularly beneficial for you.

> **Beef** - Beef shoulder roasts, chuck roasts, brisket, ground beef, sirloin, ribeyes, just to name a few. Delicious and nutritious.
>
> **Pork** - chops, roasts, loin and bacon are the cuts I eat most often.
>
> **Poultry** – I prefer the fattier cuts of poultry, the dark meats, especially thighs. I suggest eating poultry with the skin if you can. I do.

Fish – Especially fatty (oily) fish from the sea, including sardines, tuna, salmon, and mackerel.

> **Fresh Wild Caught Fish** - Unless you have sources for wild caught fish, you can try my first choice for canned seafood, Wild Planet.
>
> **Wild Game** - Wild game in general is always preferrable to factory farm meats.
>
> **Organ Meats** are particularly high in nutritional value.
>
> **Note: Organ meats** including beef liver can raise blood sugar levels. I would suggest only eating an ounce or two at a time and test your blood sugars.

Deli Meats - I eat these in a pinch, but I make sure it has -0- carbs. Check the ingredients and nutritional labels, usually roasted turkey or chicken breasts are ok.

Bone Broths - I consume bone broth often but could be consumed every day. You can purchase or make your own bone broths.

Eggs - I love and enjoy eating them in omelets and frittatas; I love them fried, scrambled, hard-boiled, poached, sunny side up, etc. Some of my favorite blog posts on eggs. Four minute eggs, Frittatas, and Omelets 101.

Vegetables – low carb fibrous greens (collards, turnip greens, spinach, kale, chard, etc), cauliflower, broccoli, green peppers, celery, cucumbers and asparagus.

Dairy - Is a special situation for many. Other than milk, which is higher in carbs, butter, ghee, cream and cheese are fine to consume daily, but you need to be careful consuming too much if your weight loss stalls.

Butter is an awesome fat to consume or cook with.

Ghee is clarified butter. You can purchase or make your own. It is a great
option for those that cannot tolerate dairy
as it is mostly animal fats.

Cream is problematic for me and for many others. IF you can limit consumption to a few tablespoons in your coffee, go for it. I cannot limit myself most of the time, so I try to avoid it except during the holidays.

Milk - AVOID ALL MILK. Raw, pasteurized, low fat, full fat... avoid it all. All milk is high carb and many are intolerant of it as well.

Most milk is in the 11 -14 grams of carbs per cup and those are just the unsweetened, non-flavored milks.

Cheese/Cream Cheese is okay as a treat or as an addition to a meal, for example, adding grated cheddar to chili is great.

But I suggest avoiding eating too much cheese, especially if you hit a weight loss stall. Just make sure to check the ingredient list and the carb totals.

Fermented Dairy - Including yogurts, kefirs, etc. YOU should only consume these if they are full fat, plain and have live active cultures. Plain means no flavoring and no added sugar. I love the unique taste of fermented dairy. Even full fat plain yogurts can be high in carbohydrates, so be careful.

Real Fats from Natural Sources – Coconut oil, real butter, ghee, virgin olive oil, avocado oil, and rendered fats such as beef, pork or poultry fats.

> **Note:** I avoid vegetable oils such as canola, peanut, safflower, soybean oil and corn oil, they are ALL inflammatory.

> They will not raise blood sugar levels immediately, but they should be avoided due to their inflammatory response in the body.

Drinks – water, tea, coffee unsweetened. No non-dairy creamers nor sweeteners should be used. I am against all sweeteners unless and until you break the grain/sugar addiction.

Condiments/Spices – Louisiana Hot Sauce, Crystals, Tabasco, Slap Ya Mama, Black and Red Pepper, Sea Salt or Himalayan Salt. (Table salt is okay but try to buy the salts mentioned). Apple Cider Vinegar with Extra Virgin Olive Oil (EVOO) makes a great salad dressing.

Once you maintain truly normal blood sugars and you break the grain, sugar and carbohydrate addictions, you can add back 'highER' carb foods, if you want to do so. Just make sure to test your blood sugars to see how your body reacts.

Foods to Consume Occasionally

Oysters/Squid – oysters and squid have carbohydrates, some oyster varieties have more than others. Pacific oysters are said to have more than Eastern varieties. You could eat these every day, but do so in small quantities (and test your blood sugars).

Organ Meats – Some organ meats (especially beef liver) can significantly raise blood sugars if too much is eaten. For this reason I usually only eat a slice (3-4 ounces) of beef liver at a time.

Alcoholic Beverages – Alcohol by itself can reduce blood sugars temporarily by blunting the liver's production of glucose. However, the problem is usually all the things that go with alcohol... the mixers. I do not consume sugary, carby mixers.

> **Mixed Drinks** - Scotch, bourbon, whisky, rum, gin, and other distilled spirits are all ok by themselves.
>
> I drink vodka sodas about once a week. It's vodka, bicarbonate water and lime juice. It's nice and 'clean'... and very low carb.
>
> **Dry Wine** - is generally low carb and ok to consume, just check the carb totals and test your blood sugars, like you should do with everything.
>
> **Low Carb Beer** - I only drink these a couple of times a year, mainly because I really prefer wine and vodka sodas. Michelob Ultra is one low carb beer that I enjoy on rare occasions, with 2.6 grams of carbs per serving. ... just watch the servings. :)

Note: Alcohol can reduce your blood sugar levels by limiting gluconeogenesis. Alcohol can also cause weight gain or a weight loss stall.

Cheese – Cheese if you can limit it's consumption, is fine to eat daily. Many people cannot and tend to over eat cheese... I am one of them. Too much cheese (or dairy in general) can for many, cause a weight loss stall or even weight gain.

Nuts – walnuts, pecans, cashews, macadamia nuts, and almonds are okay in VERY small amounts, a handful a day. I would suggest avoiding nuts until you normalize blood sugars because so many people cannot limit themselves once they start eating them. Nuts have carbs, if you do eat them, make sure to include them in your carb totals.

Fruits – Low Carb Fruits ONLY and even then, do not consume many and not daily. Avocado, blueberries, raspberries, strawberries, blackberries are fine as an occasional treat. A handful or less when consumed is advised until blood sugar is under control.

Sweeteners - I am against using sweeteners, including artificial sweeteners until the addiction to sugar and grains has been broken.

If you must, stevia, monk fruit, allulose and other artificial sweeteners can be helpful during the transitional period, but I do not recommend for long term use.

You want to break the addiction to carbohydrates including sugar, starch and grains. This is more difficult if you continue to eat sweeteners, artificial or not.

Foods to Avoid

Sugar is sugar... regardless of the source. Don't fall for the 'natural sugar' deception, that natural sugar is good for diabetics. They all raise blood sugars.

Starch is starch, regardless of the source. If it's starchy... it will spike your blood sugars.

Remember the key is to limit total carbs to 30 or less per day.

Sugar – includes soft drinks, fruit juices, cookies, cakes, muffins, candy, chocolates, confections, fruit roll-ups, sweet tea.

Avoid them all.

Starch – potatoes, beans, bread, pasta and rice are high in starches: which means they are high in carbs.

I urge you to follow my suggestion and limit total carbohydrates to 30 grams or less. Do you really want to use up 30g of carbs on one (1) potato? or exceed 30g on 1 cup of rice?

Make no mistake, eating 30g of carbs all at once will cause your blood sugars to spike, big time.

Successfully living with Type 2 diabetes is all about "rationing" carbs. By limiting the carbs to 30 grams or less you make it easier to manage blood sugars.

Grains and Cereals – Avoid grains in any form (especially glutinous wheat grains), flour, pasta, breads, crackers, cakes, cookies, cereals, corn, quinoa, oats, millet, barley and rice. - Avoid them all.

There are many reasons to avoid grains, I only need one... they are high carb and will spike blood sugars.

Vegetable and seed oils – This includes corn oil, canola oil, safflower oil, margarine, soybean oil, commercial mayonnaise, and salad dressings. Here's a post for making homemade aioli, a mayonnaise substitute and here's a post for making homemade salad dressing.

Milk - AVOID ALL MILK. Raw, pasteurized, low fat, full fat... avoid it all. All milk is high carb and many are intolerant of it as well. Most milk is in the 11 - 14g of carbs per cup and those are just the unsweetened, non-flavored milks.

Legumes – including beans and peanuts. Peanuts are technically a legume and not a nut. These are high in carbs and can be inflammatory.

High carb fruits – avoid grapes, oranges, bananas, pineapple, pears, apples and all other sweet, high carb fruits.

High carb vegetables - avoid yams, carrots, sweet potatoes, white potatoes, corn, beans, turnips, parsnips, etc.

Reduced-fat – why avoid reduced fat? Typically food companies are reducing natural fats AND they usually add sugar to compensate. These are also typically chemical laden and inflammatory. Natural fats are healthy, eat full fat natural foods.

Note: The above list may appear daunting.

** Do not try to memorize this listing before beginning.

Remember to keep it simple... especially in the beginning.

Macronutrients: Fats, Protein & Carbs

Determining your macronutrient ratios can be informative. When I first 'food journaled' (2009), it was cool to see and to compare percentages with others.

I rarely keep a food journal these days unless I am experimenting, but the results of compiling food journals since 2009 are below.

Note: Remember, you don't have to concern yourself with food journaling if you stick to the food recommendations, just make sure not to go over 30 grams of carbs, which is difficult to do if you eat only meats, cheese, eggs and leafy green vegetables.

My Historical Macronutrient Ratios

Fat 70%
Protein 28%
Carbs 2%

I have been higher and lower in each of the categories at any given time, but this is my best estimate of my typical averages.

My Personal Macronutrient Targets

Total Carbs: Less than 30 grams per day
Protein: 120 to 160 grams per day
Fats: 90 - 150 grams per day

Note:

- When I want to lose body fat, I try to stay below 100 grams of fat per day, on average.

- I am not saying these are my recommendations for you (other than carbs). Much will depend on weight, age, sex, and activity level.

  Below I explain how I came up with these numbers for me.

1. **Total Carbohydrates 30 grams or less per day**. Carbs directly affect blood sugars, keep carbs low. I suggest 30 grams of total carbohydrates or less, not 'net' carbs as some promote.

   a. I have typically eaten 5-15 g per day the last several years and I THRIVE! ... so I know 30 grams of carbohydrates, or less is more than doable.

   b. By the way, Dr. Bernstein (the preeminent diabetes specialist) promotes 30 grams per day, so that number is 'doctor approved', if that is important to you.

   c. Why total carbs instead of 'net'? Because companies will use deceptive advertising to sell products... shocking I know. Count total carbs and not 'net' carbs. Simplicity is important when first starting.

2. **Fat: I average about 150 grams of fat per day**, unless I am leaning out (losing body fat), and then I try to stay below 100 grams on average.

   Unless I am experimenting or leaning out, I do not count fat grams.

38

If you are just starting and have elevated blood sugars, concentrate on dialing in the total carbs. Nail down your blood sugars and then work on the rest. At least initially, you should lose body fat just by cutting carbs.

Fats are 'filler' for me, carbs are not a concern I just don't eat many. Protein is the only macronutrient I really worry about, I'll explain more in the next section.

3. **Protein: My goal is 120 to 160 grams per day.**

I want to consume enough to promote Muscle Protein Synthesis (MPS) for muscle growth, maintaining existing muscle and cellular repair. The range above, on average, takes care of my body's needs as a 60 year old, male diabetic.

Discussing adequate levels of protein is complicated and complex. It can vary by age, sex and overall health. Studies show that as we age, we actually need MORE protein to maintain muscle and rebuild damaged cells.

How much protein is 'enough'? Studies suggest 40 grams per meal is better than 20 grams as we age, so that's my goal as a 60 year old diabetic..

40 x 3 = 120 grams - This is the minimum on average per day. I typically only
eat twice a day so I just try to eat more when I do eat... it's not a problem for me.

160 grams - the upper end of my range. One gram of protein per pound of your ideal body weight is a good approximation.

Steve Note: We are talking averages, I am usually above the minimum but not always. Likewise, I am usually below the maximum but sometimes I go above.

I've experimented with strict carnivore diets in the past (eating nothing but animal products), the longest stint was for one full year. Based on food journals I averaged about 5 grams of total carbohydrates per day (mainly from eggs and organ meats like beef liver).

Even at this low level of carbohydrate consumption, I've seen no negative side effects, and I am still THRIVING!

Point being?

1. You can and should consume 30 grams of carbohydrates or less, at least until you obtain and maintain truly normal blood sugars.

2. Eating high protein diets are not harmful, quite the contrary, they are beneficial.

   Bonus points because you are feeding your body what it needs to build and maintain muscle, rebuild and repair cells.

Approximately how much meat is 40 grams of protein? Amounts vary but not enough to really matter, it's about 5-6 ounces of meat.

Description	Amount	Unit
Hamburger or Ground Beef, 80% Lean	6	oz
Beef Steak, Chuck, Visible Fat Eaten	6	oz
Pork Roast, Shoulder, Fresh, Visible Fat Eaten	6	oz
Pork Chops, Loin, Fresh, Visible Fat Eaten	5	oz
Chicken Thigh, Skin Eaten	5	oz
Chicken Breast, Skinless	5	oz
Salmon, Atlantic, Wild, Cooked	6	oz
Tuna, Canned, Light, Water Pack, No Salt, Drained	6	oz

Since I usually only eat twice a day, I typically will eat 10 ounces at lunch and 6 ounces at dinner. I prefer to have my larger meal at lunch and a lighter dinner.

Note: Protein amounts in this book are based on animal based proteins. The bioavailability and types of proteins vary in plant based foods, therefore I don't suggest counting plant-based foods protein grams. If you do, a rough estimate is to double the consumption of plant protein to equate with animal proteins.

Science Says: Protein Consumption

Remember the blood sugar targets and recommendations for diabetics and how wrong and harmful they are?

Too remember the carb recommendations promoted by the Medical Industry of 60 grams per meal and 15 grams of carbs for snacks...for diabetics? That totals about 225 grams of carbs per day. If I ate that many carbs, I'd still be on diabetes drugs and (4) insulin shots a day... I have no doubt.

Point Being: When I learned that the ADA and the Medical Industry would promote harmful dietary advice and harmful blood sugar targets to diabetics ... I learned to '**question everything**'.

Governmental protein recommendations are woefully low, only .8 grams of protein per kg. For me, that's only 56 grams of protein per day!

They seem to be answering the question... "What's the least amount of protein a person would need to survive?"

The question should be, "How much protein is needed to achieve optimal health and fitness?"

I've searched far and wide and found many different answers. Here's what I do know.

Protein is the most important macronutrient. Every cell in our body contains protein. It's used to rebuild and create cells... cells that include muscles, bones, blood and organs.

In this study, protein as high as 1.8 to 2.0g per kg,

"... may be advantageous in preventing lean mass losses during periods of energy restriction to promote fat loss."

Higher still, this study, 2.4g of protein was more effective than 1.2g /kg.

"Our results showed that, during a marked energy deficit, consumption of a diet containing 2.4 g protein per kg, per day was more effective than consumption of a diet containing 1.2 g protein per kg, per day in promoting increases in LBM and losses of fat mass when combined with a high volume of resistance and anaerobic exercise."

Even higher levels in another study,

"Consuming a high protein diet (3.4 g/kg/d) in conjunction with a heavy resistance-training program may confer benefits with regards to body composition. Furthermore, there is no evidence that consuming a high protein diet has any deleterious effects."

To put these in perspective, I typically eat 120 to 160 grams of protein per day. I've eaten a lot more but this is the typical range. My weight is 160 lbs or about 70 kg, so 3.4 kg per day would be well over 200 grams of protein ... and there is **no evidence** consuming over 200 grams of protein every day... is harmful.

Protein Consumption Summary

The Daily Recommended Intake (DRI) as published by the US government (.8 grams per kg) is woefully short. For me at 160 lbs that converts to about 70 kg, that would equal 56 grams of protein per day.

56 grams of protein is what I would call lunch. I've eaten much more than that per day for 13 years... and I thrive.

Protein studies (here and here), show protein needs increase as we age, not decrease. Additionally, everyone should be performing weight-resistance exercises to increase or at least maintain muscle mass.

For these reasons, I believe the average of 1 gram of protein per pound, per day, or 2.2 g per kg is wise, especially if you are trying to lose body fat.

For more information, I invite you to read this post "How Much Protein is Optimal".

However, if you have been eating very low protein, I urge you to experiment with adding protein slowly and gradually.

Note: If your blood sugars remain elevated, excess protein may be the culprit.

Experiment with reducing protein consumption, but stay above an absolute minimum of 120 grams of animal protein. Once you've obtained and maintained truly normal blood sugars you can experiment with adding more protein, once blood sugars normalize.

Weight Loss Stall

I do not believe a 'calorie is a calorie'. In other words, calories from fructose are not treated the same as calories from healthy fats or animal proteins. **This is a biological fact.**

I also do not believe the 'calories in, calories out' (CICO). By this I mean, I do not believe if you burn 7500 calories more than you consume, you will lose a pound. It depends on the macronutrients the calories come from, protein, fat, or carbs are all treated differently by the body. .

If you do not believe that all calories are treated the same in the body (they aren't) , then CICO must go.

HOWEVER, I DO BELIEVE "calories count", or more exactly, "energy counts".

Over consuming energy over an extended period of time will result in weight gain, it does for me, but the composition of those calories... (protein, fat, carbs) make a real difference in the gaining of body fat.

Many lose weight initially on a low carb diet. However for many, at some point you will need to evaluate and reduce calories to continue with your weight loss.

Why?

Since you are already low carb, and you should already be eating adequate protein... dietary fat is the place to reduce your energy (calorie) intake to restart your fat loss... in my opinion.

Just to restate for emphasis. If you reach a weight loss stall, I strongly urge you to keep a food journal for a few days, evaluate your diet and make adjustments.

Keeping a food journal can help point to areas that may need adjustments for both blood sugar levels as well as weight loss.

1. If you read the "low-carb" forums, many people have experienced 'carb creep'. Carb creep occurs by adding more and more foods that may be low in carbs but eating too much of them can add up over time.

    Nuts, some dairy (milk, etc) and fruits are the principle suspects...so keep an eye on grams of carbs.

2. Too much fat consumption can lead to body fat gains... it certainly does for me. Natural animal based fats are healthy, filling, and can help with blood sugar management... but too much, *can* lead to weight loss stalls.

3. Personally, I don't think lean proteins are a major source of weight stalls or body fat gains, at least they haven't been for me. When I want to 'lean out', I simply cut back on the high fat foods and focus on leaner cuts of meat.

    The main 'fatty foods' I cut? Sadly it's cream and cheese. I love them, but when I am attempting to lose body fat... I avoid them.

My favorite online food journal by far is Cronometer.com. It's easy to use and it's easy to plan out your day's meals as well.

Fasting / Intermittent Fasting

I am a fan of fasting and intermittent fasting ... and especially for Type 2 diabetics.

Definitions vary depending on the source but for me, fasting is when you do not consume nutrients for a 24 hour period or more.

Intermittent fasting is when you skip a meal or two.

Personally I've fasted for up to 4 days, consuming only water, but I haven't done that in years. However I do intermittent fast (skip meals) almost every day.

Note: As with any carb reduction dietary plan, check your blood sugars and adjust medications as needed.

Intermittent fasting and a truly low carb diet is POWERFUL medicine for type 2 diabetes.

Why?

I usually skip breakfast, drinking only black coffee. I then eat a heavier meal at lunch, then eat a lighter meal at dinner.

Think about this, when combined with a low carb diet, my pancreas gets to 'rest' from dinner until lunch the next day.

Compare this with the vast majority of diabetics who eat carby 'foods' from waking until bedtime. Their pancreas is overworked 24 x 7 x 365 days, it's a recipe for disaster.

And a disaster is exactly what diabetes is in 2022 ... a disaster. More and more type 2 diabetics are requiring insulin ... just to survive.

Who benefits from this scenario of diabetics eating high carb foods, maintaining harmful elevated blood sugars... and requiring more and more drugs and insulin? Not to mention the increase in doctor visits, the increase in medical device sales including Continuous Glucose Meters, Insulin Pumps, meters, etc etc.

Who benefits? Not diabetics ... the beneficiaries are the ADA, Big Food, Big Pharma and the Medical Industry.

Compare that with my story. Instead of more and more drugs and services... I weaned off drugs and insulin, and I haven't seen a doctor for diabetes or sickness since 2009. (My only medical industry contact since 2009 was following a biking accident and an emergency room visit.)

Reduced pancreatic production of insulin is common for most Type 2 diabetics due to toxic elevated blood sugars and the overworking of the pancreas.

With my meal plan and skipping a meal or two a day, my pancreas only works a few hours a day and I do not overload it with carbohydrates when I do eat.

Which makes more sense to you?

I suggest giving intermittent fasting a try 'today', but especially if your blood sugar or weight loss stalls.

Here's how I slowly implemented the strategy. Each day I delayed breakfast an hour... and I pushed lunch back an hour. In a week I was eating twice a day.

Why Fasting or Intermittent Fasting?

Carbohydrates directly increase blood sugar so you want to completely avoid them for twenty four hours.

Protein will indirectly increase blood sugar but at a much lower rate than carbohydrate.

Fats will cause minimal blood sugar increase (if any) and will provide energy for your body to function.

There are different types of fasting.

Intermittent Fasting

This is my favorite method of fasting. It's simply skipping a meal or two.

For me, I rarely eat three meals a day. I usually skip breakfast, eating only lunch and dinner. This is also called an 18/6 eating window, since I usually eat between noon and 6 PM, fasting for 18 hours a day.

As noted previously, this with a low carb diet allows my pancreas to rest for most of the day and night.

Water, Tea or Coffee Fast

True fasting is consuming no nutrients for a 24 hour period (or longer). Some go longer than 24 hours, but I do not recommend it. I have done true fasts for four days in the past, while experimenting.

So to truly 'fast' you need to consume only non-caloric drinks like water, tea and black coffee... no sweeteners or cream, of course.

I do not recommend true fasts over 24 hours, why?

I'm waging war with diabetes for the long-term.

Studies have shown muscle loss when going over 24 hours. At this stage of the game, 60 years old, I want to increase muscle mass or at least to maintain what I have.

Muscle is the single largest user of blood sugar. To help maintain normal blood sugar levels and overall health, I don't want to lose any muscle as a diabetic.

Even losing an ounce of muscle will be counterproductive. It is possible to add muscle as we age, but it takes more work as we age!

Alternate Day Fasting

Other than Intermittent Fasting, this is my recommended method of fasting.

Day 1 - eat as you normally would with adequate protein, fats and very low carb.

Day 2 - consume only water, tea or black coffee (unsweetened, no cream).

Repeat

Note: I'd suggest doing the meal plan mentioned previously (30 grams of carbs per day) for several weeks or a month first. People seem to handle fasting better when they have adjusted to low carb for at least a couple of weeks.

Also, I'd suggest trying intermittent fasting for a few weeks before fasting all day, just to make sure your body is 'ready'.

Try this for several days and pay close attention to blood sugars, making sure not to go too low.

True Fat Fasts

Ok, this isn't a "fast" in the true sense of the word. A fast is -0- nutrients for a period of time. I'm talking about eating only fats for a period of time.

A true fat fast is consuming nothing but fats, my favorites for this are butter and coconut oil. As with typical fasting, I do not recommend going over 24 hours and for the same reasons, potential muscle loss.

Therefore you should follow the "Alternate Day Fasting" rules above. Eat normally on one day and fat fast the next. Repeat if you desire.

The purpose of this is similar to typical fasting, removing the 'dietary fuel' for elevated blood sugars. The intent of consuming dietary fat is that you would help retain more muscle, as the body would have some calories for energy and would not need to break down muscle (or as much muscle).

Tips: Eat fats in small amounts, a teaspoon at a time initially. Only eat enough fat to keep you sated.
I would NOT advocate consuming vegetable or seed oils ever.

Note: When I originally did my 'fat fasts' I ate butter and coconut oil with a spoon, or just stirred it into my coffee.

However you could put a teaspoon of butter and coconut oil in a cup of black coffee. Mix and froth with a stick blender, a regular blender is fine as well.

More On Plateaus and Stalls

Okay, everything is going great. Your blood sugars are decreasing; your weight is decreasing and then suddenly, a stall or plateau.

Stalls or plateaus for a day or two are to be expected. If they persist for more than a few days, I suggest corrective action.

The first course of action could be food journaling as mentioned previously. Are you eating too many carbs, too much protein, or maybe too much fat? Check it out and make adjustments.

If that doesn't work you can try these other options.

Like anything I recommend... unless otherwise noted, I've successfully experimented with it myself.

Strict Carnivore

Strict or Full Carnivore is someone who eats all animal-based foods.

The diets may vary in strictness but the general idea is to avoid plant-based foods.

Strictest would be eating ONLY animal based foods and drinking water, with no plant-based spices and no coffee, wine or distilled spirits.

Less strict versions allow for wine, distilled spirits, coffee, teas and plant-based spices like pepper etc.

My Full Carnivore Experiment

My latest serious dietary experiment in 2017 was my version of Full Carnivore... I ate only animal based foods for a year, I did include wine, coffee and black pepper so it wasn't as strict as some.

But it was an outstanding success! After an entire year of almost zero carb... I felt great. No negative repercussions at all from eating no fiber from plants for an entire year.

It was so successful, I added it to this book.

For me and for most of the people I have helped, breaking the addictions to grains and sugar is the most difficult part of eating this way and can take one to three months. Sadly, many fail and suffer from wave after wave of diabetic complications.

If you have difficulty breaking addictions and keep 'falling off the wagon', ... I urge you to give 'full-carnivore' a try. It's very simple.

Eat only animal based foods, beef, pork, fish, poultry, cheese and eggs.

There are many reports of people breaking addictions to carbs (grains and sugar) when they had failed before, by eating a 'full carnivore', all-meat diet.

Once you break the addictions, you can go back to eating 30 grams of carbohydrate per day, or not.

The more I eat only meat... the more I only want meat to eat. Give it a try for 30 days! ... It can change your life. You can read more about my experience with a Carnivore Diet, "Diabetic Carnivore" and "Summary".

As with any low carb diet, you will need to monitor your blood glucose as you crank down the carbs... and your blood sugars begin to drop.

I began to reduce my medications and insulin as my fasting blood sugars began to sink into normal, non-diabetic range... HEY, that's a beautiful thing!! Rejoice!

If you are unsure, contact your physician. I stopped all diabetes drugs and insulin when my Fasting Blood Sugars were consistently in the sub 90 mg/dl (5.0 mmol/l) range.

Snacks

I'm about to start my 14th year with diabetes... I like to only eat twice a day.

That's two meals and -0- snacking. That may be **SHOCKING** to some ... that's ok, it would have been shocking to me as an obese, chronically sick... and constantly snacking diabetic.

When you first start eating low carb, you absolutely want to snack... if you feel hungry, but you need to snack on low carb foods always.

You do not want to go hungry, that opens the door for caving in and eating high carb, sugary, glutenous 'junk'.

So when you first start, you need to make sure you have plenty of low carb snacks available.

Road Warrior Snacks

These are snacks you can toss in the glove compartment, briefcase or lunch box.

1. **Canned fish** - including sardines, tuna, salmon, herring, mackerel, etc. True story, I kept cans of sardines and mackerel with a can-opener in my glove compartment for YEARS just in case of an emergency.

2. **Pork skins, pork rinds, bacon puffs etc.** - Check the ingredients for carbs of course but I like to buy the ones that just have 'salt and pork'. Here's a post on pork rinds.

3. **Canned Meats** - There are canned chicken, beef, pork etc ... it's been over a decade since I've looked at these, just check the ingredients carefully... I really like to avoid any additives. I'd only buy them if the ingredients were meat and spices like salt and packed in water or broth.

4. **Nuts** - be careful with these. I love nuts... but I love them too much. I'd carry only single servings for emergencies, an ounce or two. Pecans are my favorite from a cost and macronutrient profile, they are relatively low in carbs.

5. **Avocados** - you can't toss these in the back seat and forget about them, but these will keep for days especially if 'uncut' and they are purchased green and hard. When it's time to eat, just halve them and remove the pit. The outer shell makes a nice 'bowl'. :)

Note: There are many new 'low carb' and 'keto' snacks on the market today. I've had very little experience with them. Some are good, but many are not so if you want to experiment with these snacks, tread lightly and test them against your meter.

I'd suggest waiting until after you obtain normal blood sugars and after you have broken the carb/grain addictions before trying them.

Snacks with a Shorter Shelf Life

These are snacks with a shorter 'shelf life' than canned sardines. :)

Note: You can include any food that is listed in the "Foods" section earlier in the book.

1. **Boiled eggs** - especially left in their shell, make great travel snacks.

2. **Bacon, turkey, chicken, roast beef** etc - I've cooked all of these the night before and taken with me on all-day trips, tossing them in a cooler.

3. **Cheeses** - cheddar, cottage cheese, cream cheese, etc - great in combination with any of the above items... or alone.

4. **Vegetables** - unsweetened pickles, celery, cucumbers, broccoli, zucchini, cauliflower, etc.

In a Pinch

There really is no excuse for 'cheating'.

But let's say you are on the road without any low carb snacks... what to do?

1. **Fast Food Restaurants:** I've ordered bunless burgers at many fast food restaurants. And I've ordered just 'burger patties' at Hardees, Wendy's, McDonald's and Burger King.

You may have to explain it to the person at the register but there are 'side order' patties at most (if not all) fast food restaurants.

2. **Formal Restaurants:** Most restaurants will allow you to order bunless burgers, or to substitute steamed vegetables (usually broccoli and cauliflower) for potatoes.

3. **Grocery Stores:** I've made quick stops to buy rotisserie chicken, roast beef, turkey, or chicken. Just make sure they are 'low carb' deli meats. Always check the ingredients added to the meats.

When I eat, I try to eat until I'm no longer hungry. I try NOT to stuff myself... but I want to eat enough when I do eat, to keep me satisfied and to keep me from snacking.

Point Being: If you feel the urge to snack between meals, you may simply need to eat more at your meals.

Once I adapted to a low carb diet (it took a couple of weeks), I began cutting back on snacking. I've mentioned why earlier, but to restate it here... I want to rest my pancreas as much as possible.

We'll move on to exercise.

Exercise

All movement, all exercise is good, assuming it's done properly.

But not all exercise is good for diabetics ... all the time.

Best Exercises for Blood Sugar Reduction

Slow and steady exercises are generally excellent for reducing blood sugars.

Walking: The single most popular exercise for reducing blood sugars immediately is walking. Below are other exercises for helping to reduce blood sugars.

Knee Raises: Knee raises are basically 'walking in place' and if done methodically as if walking, are great for knocking down blood sugars. If you can't go outside for a walk, standing knee raises are a good option you can do anywhere.

Bicycling at a low or slow rate is also excellent exercise for reducing blood sugars. It's also low impact, which is great for some people with joint pain. Bicycling can be done intensely. I love sprinting on bicycles, but if my blood sugars are elevated, I bike around the neighborhood very slowly with a nice, steady pace.

Push Mowing the Yard - this is actually my all-time favorite blood sugar reducing exercise. I've tested this many times and it works for me... every single time. I don't try to push fast or too hard... just taking my time, push-mowing my lawn.

Anaerobic vs Aerobic

Anaerobic means 'without oxygen'. When the exercise becomes so intense that you can't easily talk or catch your breath... that's anaerobic or intense exercise.

Very intense exercise almost always spikes my blood sugars. I've had spikes of 30-40 points mg/dl (2-2.5 mmol/l) after 'Maximum Jump Burpees' as well as after "Maximum 55 lb kettlebell swings". Another one of my favorite 'very intense' exercises is sprints and yes, they spike my blood sugars as well.

With very intense exercise, the spike can hit hard and fast... as if I'd eaten sugar or grains. I love highly intense exercise but if my blood sugars are over 100 mg/dl, I won't do highly anaerobic, highly intense exercises.

Note: As we know walking (or any low intensity exercise) is awesome for reducing blood sugars, and this includes after performing intense exercise.

I love intense exercise, just not if my blood sugars are elevated. I wrote a post about this, "Diabetes and Exercise".

On the next page is a chart from that post. I tested my blood sugars with a CGM while performing three very intense exercises.

1. Maximum Kettlebells in 15 minutes, these 'jacked' my blood sugars as fast as eating pure sugar.

2. Maximum Jump Burpees jacked my blood sugars even higher, but took a little longer to spike and to return to normal.

3. Intense Cardio also raised my blood sugars, but not to the extent of the others.

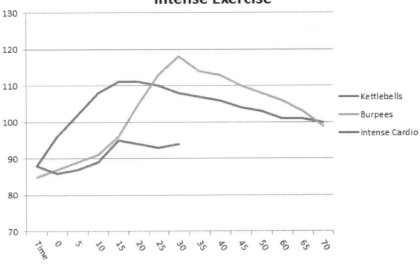

Blood Sugars and Intense Exercise

Kettlebells
Burpees
Intense Cardio

Starting an Exercise Routine

I love telling the story. When I arrived home from the hospital as a freshly diagnosed diabetic, I began working out with my wife's aerobic weights... 8 lbs dumbbells.

Back then walking to the mailbox was all the exercise I could handle at one time... I was in terrible 'shape', I was obese and very lethargic.

But after the big "D" diagnosis, I was committed to improving my health and fitness so I sucked it up... and my first 'workout' was literally walking to the very next mailbox on my street.

The next day and subsequent days, I would continue walking to the next mailbox, and the next day to the next mailbox, etc. After a while, I even brought along the aerobic weights to curl and overhead press as I walked.

59

Once I could walk a mile, I began to alternate walking and jogging. Next I alternated jogging and running a mile. Once I could run a mile, I began adding distance, eventually I worked my way up to running 10.2 miles every other day.

At that point, I realized that I needed to add strength and began adding in more weight resistance training in earnest.

Point Being: Do NOT be ashamed if you can not walk or jog very far. I know what it is like... just push through it and do a little more each day.

In other words, today, do what you can do comfortably... and try to do a little more tomorrow, and the next day, and the day after that.

My Exercise Routine Today

Most days a week (5-6 days) I perform weight resistance, it's usually bodyweight exercises... push ups, squats, and pull ups.

Depending on how I feel I'll add in curls, shrugs, and various dumbbell exercises.

If you don't have equipment and don't want to spend a lot of money upfront, try purchasing a suspension trainer from Walmart or Amazon. I bought a simple one for less than $20. It's awesome for doing workouts in the home attached to a door... or tied to a tree for an outside workout.

It's important to perform some type of exercise every day. You may have to start out doing push ups on your knees or leaning over a table, etc ... the main thing is to move every day and if you can perform some type of weight resistance, even better!

Note: Check with your doctor before starting any exercise routine. The key with any workout or exercise program is to ... HAVE FUN!

Do exercises you enjoy!

Here are more posts on some of the exercises I've performed over the years. I went from barely being able to walk to the next mailbox to ... LOVING intense exercise.

Are You Sure You Are Ok?
Triple 100 for 30 Days - Daily Pushups, Pullups, and Squats
1,058 Pushups in a Day
35 Minutes of Hell
Intense Exercise Experiments
Diabetes and Barefoot Exercise

Next we'll move to supplements.

Nutritional Supplements

First let's talk about supplements in general and then we'll talk about supplements for diabetes specifically.

General Supplements

Vitamin D3 - It's the only supplement I take every day, 10,000 IU daily.

I'm a strong believer in D3 supplementation for everyone, studies show the vast majority of people are woefully deficient. Unless you live near the equator and work outside in shorts most of the day, I think everyone should supplement D3.

As we age people need to supplement vitamin D3 more... not less. Studies show our bodies process less D3 from sunlight as we age.

Most studies suggest that supplementation of 5,000 IU per day is a safe number, but just so you know, I take 10,000 IU per day living in the northern latitudes. Living in Canada, we only get D3 from the sun in significant amounts during the summer.

You could get your D3 level checked, reputable sources I trust suggest 50-80 ng/ml is an optimum range.

Potassium - I supplement occasionally with "NoSalt" which is Potassium Chloride. I just sprinkle some on my food periodically.

Magnesium - Magnesium is a very important mineral, I know people who take it every day and have done so for years. I take it but typically only a few times a week.

Low Carb or Keto Flu: Especially when starting low carb you can suffer from what is called low carb or keto 'flu' as your body adjusts. Three supplements can help tremendously with your body's adjustment period... magnesium, potassium and salt.

I don't use these products, but if you'd prefer to take one supplement for magnesium, potassium and sodium there are two products I recommend, **LMNT Keto Electrolyte Powder and Snake Juice Electrolyte Packs**

Supplements for Blood Sugar Control

I will not get into dosing levels but I will list supplements that people have used and reported improved blood sugars. These results are from people that I know and trust, or supplements that I've used.

Note: By the time I began experimenting with supplements for blood sugar reduction, I had already achieved truly normal blood sugars. Therefore when I experimented with the supplements, my response might have been less than someone with elevated blood sugars.

Point Being: Your results may and probably will differ from my own experience.

I tested these supplements with little effect but have heard good things about them from others: Iodine, Apple Cider Vinegar, Chromium and Cinnamon.

I've heard good things about alpha lipoic acid (ALA), Biotin, Berberine, and Insulow but I have not tried them.

Check with a trusted source to make sure there are no drug interactions with the supplements if you try them. If you do not have a trusted source, check with your medical industry professional. :)

Diabetes Drugs or Insulin

You need to obtain normal blood sugars. If diet, supplementation and exercise is not enough there is no shame in taking a diabetic drug or insulin.

The key to a path toward better health and fitness is to achieve normal blood sugars, by any means necessary. Regardless, you should always eat a low-carb meal plan in my opinion.

When I was first diagnosed I was on Actos AND two insulins (four shots a day). It's my opinion that insulin was especially important for my recovery. I had been horrendously over-working my pancreas and it needed a rest.

Injecting insulin and ratcheting down the carbohydrates allowed my pancreas to rest and 'restart'. I was originally diagnosed as a Type 1 diabetic.

If you have to take a diabetes drug, just do your research and avoid those with harmful side effects. **Metformin and Metformin ER** (for those that have stomach issues), are the drugs that several of my friends have used, and continue to use with success.

With insulin and a low carb diet I quickly obtained normal blood sugars. As my pancreas started picking up the slack, I began to reduce my insulin until one day I didn't need it anymore... I didn't need drugs nor insulin anymore.

The rest as they say ... is history!

Do NOT be ashamed to take insulin or diabetes drugs.

Try your best to live without them, but in the end, the MAIN goal is to obtain and maintain truly normal blood sugars!

**Important: Please, I urge you… don't rely on drugs alone to attempt to reduce your blood sugars into normal ranges. You are here reading this book because eating a high carb diet and taking drugs… failed miserably.

"Carb up and shoot up" is a failed long term diabetes treatment strategy.

Follow a very low carb diet, exercise daily and if that doesn't work, then look at medications or insulin.

It's Now Up to You

I've shown you a better way to help control your blood sugars and to lose weight.

I've shown you a way to break through weight loss stalls and plateauing of blood sugars.

I've given you my blood sugar targets with the evidence I used to justify them. (more in the Addendum)

I've given you simple exercises to improve your blood sugars and your fitness.

I have given you suggestions on supplements, drugs and insulin to help control your blood sugars should diet and exercise not be enough.

NOW it's up to you!

Recommended Next Steps

Here are the steps... to reclaim your life and your health.

1. Go grocery shopping for meats, leafy green or fibrous vegetables, eggs, and cheese.

2. Throw everything away that is not mentioned in #1.

I am very serious, the best thing you can do today is to throw out all of the high carb foods listed in the "Foods to Avoid" section. Get rid of all of the temptations.

However, I know it's difficult if there are others in the home who won't be eating as you. Therefore step #2 is optional, if you live with others, but Step #1 is not.

But you need to decide to start the diet section ....TODAY!

Not tomorrow... not next week... today!

Tip: Cook meats, vegetables and eggs in large batches using broiler pans, crock pots or even grills. Freeze leftovers into separate meal servings.

You are on your way!

Relax, take deep breaths and go for a walk. Your journey to improved health and fitness has begun!! Soon you will be adding years to your life and adding life to your years!

Bonus Tip: Use your favorite search engine and type this in, with your favorite meals.

"Low Carb Alternative to _____"

Do this for all of your favorite foods.

Most of the pain and suffering caused by Type 2 diabetes could be prevented if people would simply look for low carb alternatives to their favorite foods!

Better yet, just eat like I do... meats, fibrous vegetables, cheese, eggs, and the occasional nuts and berries.

Wishing you all much success and .... TRULY NORMAL BLOOD SUGARS!

Additional Food Links

Diabetic Friendly Recipes
A Meal Plan You Can "Live With"
Sample Diabetes Meal Plan
Diabetic Nutritional Chart

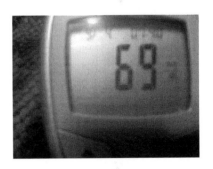

Addendum: My Blood Sugar Targets

Just to restate my personal goals ...

Preferred Overnight Fasting Blood Sugar Goals = 70 - 90 mg/dl.

Sub 100 mg/dl (5.5 mmol/l) all the time except for occasional and brief visits into the 120 mg/dl range (6.6 mmol/l) post intense exercise.

I like to stay below 100 all the time but temporary, occasional trips to 120 mg/dl (6.6 mmol/l) are ok in my opinion.

Notes:

I really do not want to exceed 100 mg/dl (5.5 mmol/l) but I know that I will occasionally and I am okay with that as long as it's occasional and the time above 100 mg/dl (5.5 mmol/l) is brief.

Most medical industry professionals will differ from my targets. Their ranges will be anywhere from 70-139 mg/dl (3.8 - 7.7 mmol/l) fasting and 140 to 180 mg/dl (7.7 - 10 mmol/l) one or two hours post meal.

Harmful vs Healthy Blood Sugars

I share with you the science and studies about the risks of elevated blood sugars.

Blood Sugar Levels and Dementia

According to this American Academy of Neurology 2013 study lower blood sugars are better for the brain. Keep in mind the study subjects were NOT diabetic nor were they pre-diabetic. The study also excluded people who were overweight or who drank more than 3.5 servings of alcohol per day.

"Our results indicate that even in the absence of manifest type 2 diabetes mellitus or impaired glucose tolerance, chronically higher blood glucose levels exert a negative influence on cognition, possibly mediated by structural changes in learning-relevant brain areas. Therefore, strategies aimed at lowering glucose levels even in the normal range may beneficially influence cognition in the older population, a hypothesis to be examined in future interventional trials."

Did you get that? EVEN people in the upper ranges of normal blood sugars have cognitive decline.

Higher Blood Sugars and the Brain

In a study also from the American Academy of Neurology, looks at the effect of blood sugars that were on the high end of normal ranges.

"People whose blood sugar is on the high end of the normal range may be at greater risk of brain shrinkage that occurs with aging and diseases such as dementia"

"After controlling for age, high blood pressure, smoking, alcohol use and other factors, the researchers found that blood sugar on the high end of normal accounted for six to 10 percent of the brain shrinkage."

Still MORE evidence elevated 'normal' blood sugars increase the risk of dementia.

Dementia risk tied to blood sugar level, even with no diabetes

"A Joint Group Health-University of Washington (UW) study in the New England Journal of Medicine has found that higher blood sugar levels are associated with higher dementia risk, even among people who do not have diabetes."

Translation: Even non-diabetics with 'higher' blood sugar have higher risk of dementia.

If higher blood sugar damages the brain causing dementia in non-diabetics, why in the hell would anyone else promote 'targets' that are above non-diabetic normal ranges? Yet people in the medical industry do promote 'above normal' goals and ranges for diabetics.

" ... in people without diabetes, risk for dementia was 18 percent higher for people with an average glucose level of 115 milligrams per deciliter compared to those with an average glucose level of 100 mg/dl."

In people with blood sugar averaging 115 mg/dl (6.3 mmol/l) the risk for dementia was 18% higher than for those who averaged 100 mg/dl (5.5 mmol/l)!! Just so you know, that is pre-diabetic blood sugar ranges.

I want to stay BELOW 100 mg/dl (5.5 mmol/l) as much as I can, obviously above 100 mg/dl is not advantageous to brain cells.

Blood Sugar Levels and Pancreatic Damage

In this study, they looked at subjects who had fasting normal blood sugars and compared pancreatic function with people with higher and higher blood sugar levels.
The threshold for truly normal blood sugars was 99 mg/dl or 5.5 mmol/l.

Below that number there was less LOSS of pancreatic function. The higher you went above that number, there was progressively MORE LOSS of pancreatic function.

People with blood sugars in normal but at the higher range of normal blood sugars, the pancreas begins a progressive decline in beta-cell function... the higher the blood sugars rise.

This study highlights why so many diabetics are requiring insulin pumps and continuous glucose monitors to 'survive'.

The overwhelming majority of diabetics eat a high carb diet and maintain elevated pre-diabetic and diabetic levels of blood sugars. It's toxic to the pancreas even in elevated but still within normal ranges.

That's why it is so damn important to maintain TRULY normal blood sugars ... and remember, elevated blood sugars are toxic to every cell and organ in the body.

Here's a study on All-Cause Mortality and A1C

Patients in the highest quartile of A1Cs were more than twice as likely to die than those in the lowest quartile.

"A greater variability in HbA1C was associated with elevated risk of mortality. Our findings underscore the need to achieve normal and consistent glycemic control to improve clinical outcomes among individuals with type 2 diabetes."

A1C and Cardiovascular Events

In this study, variation of A1c levels was independently associated with the development of major cardiovascular events in patients with type 2 diabetes and multivessel CAD during a long-term follow-up period.

"The results showed that a 1-point increase in A1c values was independently associated with a 22% increase in the risk of the combined end point of death, MI, or ischemic stroke."

Study: Blood Sugars of Healthy People

I love this next study, I saved it for last. Sadly this study is no longer available online, so I can't provide a link.

The study concerns non-diabetics and the effect of high carb meals on their blood sugars. They do not state what the high carb meals were, only that they were high carb.

Note: For most humans in the western world eating high carb foods begins almost at birth. Even if babies are breastfed the carbs come piling in soon enough... with 'cereals', mashed fruit, fruit juices, then graduating to pancakes, waffles, buns, muffins, and more cereals.

Point Being: Early on we are fed high carb, sugary, glutenous 'food' which jacks our blood sugars and insulin. Insulin resistance is a continuum and starts years and decades before a disease diagnosis... meaning people are 'abnormal' long before an official diagnosis.

The subjects in the study below were supposedly healthy.

This term is often used in error. A lack of a disease diagnosis doesn't mean healthy. These subjects shouldn't be deemed healthy just because they haven't been diagnosed with diabetes (or any disease).

Proof of what I say is in a study a couple of years ago, stating that approximately 88% of Americans are metabolically unhealthy.

Just keep this in mind. These 'healthy' people likely had metabolic damage, the level of damage had not manifested itself ... yet.

The Study

Note: I hate not being able to share the link to this study, but it's an important study, so I'm sharing it anyway. (see next page)

The average non-diabetic person spends more than 80% of their time below 100 mg/dl (5.5 mmol/l) and spends about 95% of their time below 120 mg/dl (6.6 mmol/l).

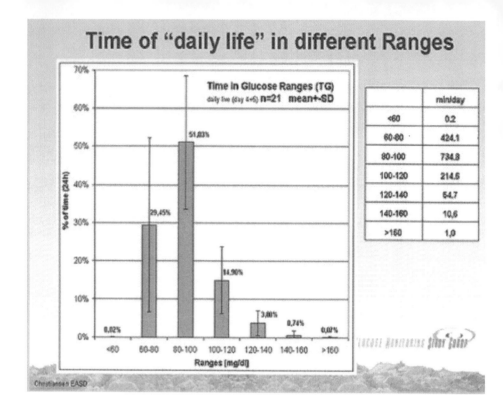

Looking at the next graph (next page), it shows the same information in a different way.

Non-diabetics even eating a high carb meal spend very little time above 100 mg/dl.

In this study, they typically start around 80 mg/dl, spike during the high carb meal but quickly come back into the sub 100 mg/dl.

From the chart we can see that non-diabetics are typically below 100 mg/dl (5.5 mmol/l) two hours after a meal.

This study and all of the other science papers and studies should be enough to convince anyone…

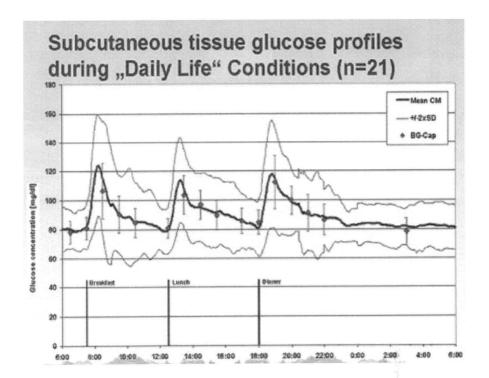

If you want to avoid diabetic complications, if you want to live a life without the anxiety of looming health conditions caused by diabetes and insulin resistance... the path should be clear.

Obtain and maintain TRULY normal blood sugars.

Addendum Summary

Study after study points in the same general direction.

The blood sugar ranges promoted by the ADA and the medical industry are wrong.

Study after study proves above 'normal' blood sugars were associated with dementia, reduced brain function, cell and organ damage.

Truly normal blood sugar ranges are therapeutic or at least neutral and would allow the body to attempt to heal itself and not to continue to cause more health problems.

Fasting blood sugars over 100 mg/dl (5.5 mmol/l) are associated with increased risk for dementia, reduced brain function, cell, and organ damage.

Healthy non-diabetics spend little time above 100 mg/dl, **even** after high carb meals.

Given all of the information I set my targets at 70-90 mg/dl. (3.8 to 5.0 mmol/L).

That way, if I 'miss the mark' a little I'll still be below 100 mg/dl (5.5 mmol/L) where the damage apparently begins. (Although we know that some damage begins even at higher levels of normal blood sugars.)

When it comes to maintaining proper health, especially when it has to do with diabetes and diabetic complications, I prefer a **"better safe than sorry approach"**.

The Medical Industry's approach causes more cell and organ

damage, requiring more drugs and more medical industry services. Coincidence?

I am in the best health of my adult life and I take no drugs and need no medical industry services. I am THRIVING and not just surviving!

Best of all, I live diabetic complication... FREE!!!

Won't you join me with reclaiming your ZEST FOR LIVING?!

We need more Diabetes Warriors!

What are you waiting for ...

GET BUSY!

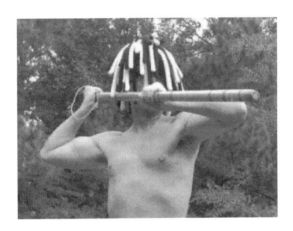

Made in the USA
Middletown, DE
29 November 2022

16325022R00047